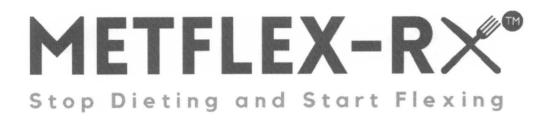

METFLEX-RX™
Stop Dieting and Start Flexing

The Ultimate Fat Loss Guide

D1455960

By Tommy Caldwell

TABLE OF CONTENTS

INTRODUCTION   2

ABOUT THE AUTHOR   5

METFLEX-RX PRINCIPLES   8

THE METFLEX-RX FUNDAMENTALS   20

THE DETAILS OF THE DIET   32

STRATEGIES AND TACTICS   56

BEHAVIOUR CHANGE   64

SUPPLEMENTATION   78

CLOSING THOUGHTS   85

REFERENCES   87

INTRODUCTION

Thousands of 'weight loss' books are published each year, and the fitness industry gets increasingly confusing. Some 'professionals' suggest that you omit entire food groups like Vegan and Carnivore authors. Others demonize whole macronutrients like fat or carbohydrate. The remainder of diet publications can only be described as insane gimmicks, like eating 30 bananas per day or just potatoes. Like most needlessly complex matters in life, there are grains of truth everywhere, but what is optimal is located somewhere in the middle.

Why does every diet need to have a 'hook'? Popular diets are a matter of 'just eat this' and 'don' t eat that' or filled with magic foods that you can't convert into body fat. If you want to make a splash in the noisy world of weight loss, you must propose a bold solution to a difficult problem. The simpler you make the issue of weight loss sound, the more clicks and purchases you'll get. We love concepts that open with 'all you have to do is stop/start eating 'x'! As readers, we want the answer to our complex weight problems to be simple, and the more outrageous the suggestion, the more likely we are to give it a try.

I am here to tell you what other authors and authorities in the industry won't. Weight loss and the achievement of any significant fitness goal is not an easy feat. Transformation won't happen quickly, and if it does, you are much more likely to relapse and regain whatever weight you have lost. Weight loss is complex, and there are many variables you must address outside of diet and exercise if you want to succeed in the long run. Weight loss is highly individual.

While there are many commonalities to be found between the general population's successes, a cookie-cutter approach to diet and exercise is not likely to work for you. Lastly, the simple, boring, daily choices you already know you should be making are where 90% of your progress will come. We are always looking for the 10% in supplements, fads, trends, and gimmicks to make up for the 90% contributors that we already understand to be the difference makers.

This book is about the 90%. It's about the daily, individual choices you need to make in your diet over time to reach your goals. There aren't any tricks, secrets, or magic to be found here. Just the hard truth.

I'm not implying that there aren't methods to be learned or strategies to be applied. In this book, you will learn about helpful foods, serving sizes, nutrient timing, behaviour change, and a few other useful techniques to maximize your results, but they stem from the absolute basics. My goal is to teach you the fundamentals of nutrition that you can apply to your unique situation to move forward in your weight loss journey confidently.

What makes this diet stand out is:

A- There isn't any dogma or ideology behind this diet. I'm not trying to get famous or feel important with what I have written. I want to help you get past the B.S. and succeed. I provide simple, proven methods that lead to the most consistent results.

B- There isn't any food group or nutrient demonization found in these pages. Some foods work well for some while the same foods can be problematic for others. Aside from obvious junk, 'good' vs. 'bad' food is not as clear as some would lead you to believe. I will show you how to navigate the best choices for you, the individual.

C- I teach the strategies that increase metabolic Flexibility using various foods, which is the key to long-term health goals. That is not a gimmick. I did not create the concept of Metabolic Flexibility, and I'm not attempting to market it. Metabolic Flexibility is simply the core philosophy of this way of eating.

I encourage you to read along and embrace this simple way of eating. If you use the tools and resources I have provided to stay consistent, you will reach your goal, and you will do so on your terms with the least amount of resistance possible. It won't be easy, but the process will be straightforward, and you will find various means of support throughout the book.

Enjoy

ABOUT THE AUTHOR

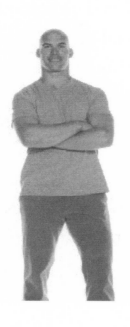

With so many people in the nutrition space, it can be challenging to decide if a dietary approach is right for you. It is difficult to trust the nutritional advice that a professional may suggest because there is so much misinformation in the world. The dietary landscape has become incredibly confusing. The best I can do is tell you a bit about myself, my history, and my approach, and then you can decide if you want to trust me with your health.

I started working in the fitness industry in 2008. Initially, I worked with high-level athletes. I have worked with players from Team Canada Hockey, Rugby Canada, the Russian World Junior Gold Medal Team, and the German World Junior Team (to name a few). I have also consulted for a variety of other sports teams and educational institutions since that time. Working with athletes was highly rewarding for me. It forced me to think critically about what I programmed for my clients doing and why. Still, at some point, I realized that most athletes will be healthy with or without me. When you are being paid to compete at the highest level, diet and exercise typically aren't a struggle for you. I wanted to put my efforts and skills toward demographics that could use my expertise in life-changing ways.

In 2011, I opened Hybrid Fitness: a gym for the average person who is looking to lose weight, increase energy, and be the healthiest version of him or herself. Since that time, I have helped thousands of everyday people to lose weight, perform better, and take control of their health. The successful approach I use with my clients is what you will find in this book.

I have accreditations in Sports Nutrition and Sport Psychology, Counseling, and Cognitive Behavioral Therapy. I have also attained my Masters in Business and continue my education with mentorship programs and other relevant coursework. Most importantly, I care about the people I work with, and I do my best every day to make a difference. This my life's work, and I take this responsibility very seriously. I hope you will trust me with your health and continue with this book as I know the information inside will guide you toward your goals.

Previous Writings

In addition to what I've noted in my bio, I wrote a bestselling behavior change book titled 'Heavy Brain.'The book culminated in everything I have learned over the years regarding why we struggle to make healthy decisions. I have a unique perspective and skillset in this area.

I am formally trained in counseling, CBT, CI, and other areas of behavioral psychology. My training in this area has left me with a unique perspective on why it is so difficult for the average person to make healthy decisions. In Heavy Brain, I detail the process of taking control in this critical area. Over 10,000 people to date have read my book. I am proud of the concepts I created and how the book has influenced readers' lives. Those who understand the Heavy Brain principles will have a much easier time applying the dietary advice delivered in this book. Reading my first book is not critical for succeeding with this diet, but it will certainly help you make the principles 'stick'.

METFLEX-RX PRINCIPLES

Before getting into the MetFlex-Rx Diet details, I would like to give you a high-level overview of the approach. Doing so will help you understand my personal philosophy on health and how it has shaped this book.

Principle 1: Create a metabolically flexible environment

Some of us struggle to maintain healthy blood sugar and insulin levels. Many of us are inefficient fat burners. A metabolically flexible person can use both carbohydrates and fats as needed to fuel the demands of their body. Suppose you want to burn fat, manage blood sugar levels, and be fit. In that case, you must be able to effectively use a variety of energy sources. If you struggle to metabolize fat, you will suffer. If you struggle to metabolize carbohydrates, you will also hit roadblocks. The way 'experts' have attempted to deal with this issue in the past is by demonizing entire nutrient categories or food groups.

In the '70s, fat became public enemy number one, a shift influenced by the sugar industry. As we broke into the new Millennium, carbohydrates started to become the latest food evil. This wasn't just the case for sugar, but carbohydrates as a whole. All along the way, we have blamed protein for everything from kidney disease to cancer. What's left to eat?

Here's the truth: 'Carbs' are not bad. Fat is not harmful. Protein is safe and effective, even in high doses. Red meat, dairy, fruit, and other whole foods that have recently become controversial should not be off-limits for all people.

Suppose you understand how to make nutrition work for you and why you should include or avoid certain foods on an individual level. In that case, you can ignore 'black and white' dietary advice. As long as you are eating a whole food diet and avoiding the obvious junk, success is much more about making your food work for you. Acting as an individual is key to positive health outcomes. Individuality is challenging to implement in the era of diet tribes.

When you are metabolically flexible, you can use both carbohydrates and fats as needed to serve your body. You can stop obsessing over 1% of dietary issues and focus on the high-impact actions that make the difference in your health. You will finally create an efficient internal state, which results in greater energy, significant fat loss potential, and increased performance.

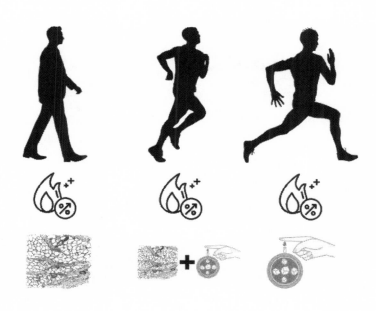

At rest, we primarily metabolize fat. As our energy demands rise, we shift toward using more glucose, yet still a mix of both substrates. At the highest intensity exercise we use primarily glucose.

Principle 2: Be Flexible in Philosophy

The world of nutrition is currently in a war. Most expert advice comes from a place of emotion and ideology rather than a place of open questioning and critical thinking. Paleo, Carnivore, Keto, and Plant-Based communities (to name a few) are tribal and hostile rather than honest and helpful. It has become more important to be on a dietary team than to do what is best for your body. The MetFlex-Rx approach doesn't have a 'team' or a box you must fit inside. Consider MetFlex the 'choose your own adventure' of diet guides.

I ask that you drop your preconceived notions about nutrition and be open to changing your mind about your current beliefs. I also ask that you resist turning the MetFlex-Rx approach into another diet identity. You are not your diet. The way you eat should serve you and your goals, not signal your diet tribe that you're part of the group. Groups don't get to the truth; they merely get to a consensus. I am offering you a simple framework to help you understand how to make many foods work for your body. Leave the dogma elsewhere, and I promise to do so as well.

Principle 3: Be Flexible in Your Expectations

If your single motivation for picking up this guide is so you can lose 20 pounds in 20 days, you will fail. You could probably lose weight quickly if you really wanted to, but could you keep it off? I doubt it. Arbitrary expectations are a promise to suffer in the future. The 'I need results now' mentality has never served you, and it isn't going to help you now. Your body is not your slave, and it will not change based on your expectations.

That is not to say that you shouldn't have goals. But your superficial goal should not be your central focus. If the only way you measure your success is with a scale, it may serve you in the short term, but it will crush you in the long run. What you should be obsessing over is your process. For example, suppose you are 50lbs overweight. In that case, there are specific actions you've taken too frequently (like snacking) and activities you've performed to rarely (like exercise). If you're like most people, you have a mix of bad habits you need to reduce and good habits you need to increase. Making the necessary changes in these areas is what is going to lead to your success.

You should become 'action-centric,' and actions are what you should measure. If you eat takeout every night of the week, can you reduce that number to three or four nights of eating out? If you can do so consistently, the weight will come off, and you will move toward your goal. If instead, you spend each morning staring at your scale, you will become frustrated and lose focus on what matters. You are going to go off track. You are going to eat food that you shouldn't eat. You are going to gain some weight back after you lose some. If you are rigid in your expectations, you will feel like a failure and sabotage yourself every time you judge your success on pure metrics.

Those who win the fitness game are the ones who can stay positive long enough to see some legitimate results. Becoming action-centric is the simplest way to achieve this resilient mindset.

Most of us are so goal obsessed that we become psychologically defeated before we ever get over the hump and into the resilience stage. Focus on your trajectory in a non-specific way and remember that the consistency of small, meaningful changes is what drives success. You want to focus on lead measures (the actions), not lag measures (what the scale says).

LEAD MEASURES

- How many times you exercise each week.
- How many of your own meals you make
- How much sleep you get each night
- How many alcoholic beverages you drink in a week
- How often you eat dessert or snack foods

LAG MEASURES

- How much weight you have lost
- The change in your pant size
- How your figure looks in the mirror
- Your body fat percentage
- The inches measured on your waist

Actions

Outcomes

If you change your behavior, you change your body. If you only focus on improving your body, your behavior never changes. This is why most of us quit before getting over the hump.

This diet is not for the desperate. The MetFlex-Rx approach is for those who are tired of failing and committed to doing what it takes to be healthy. Whether that takes one year, five years, or a decade to achieve. "Wait a decade to see results? Are you crazy?" If this is how you feel about investing your body, I've got news for you: Time is going to pass whether you like it or not. You can be fit in 10 years, or you can be sick and obese a decade from now. Today's attitude will determine which direction you continue to move in. Wouldn't you rather just be healthier when it's all said and done? Remove your rigid expectations, and you'll get where you want to go, and you'll get to your goal in the most efficient way.

Common Problems with Dietary Approaches

In this section, I will review the common issues that I see in most traditional dietary approaches. It is essential to understand why the paths you have followed in the past have not worked for you. Below is an outline of how I have accounted for these problems in this book.

Diet or Dogma?

I don't care much for the traditional structure of 'diets.' My dislike for the terminology pushed me to initially removed the word 'diet' from the MetFlex-Rx title. As much as I dislike the implications of terms like 'dieting,' it is a word that we universally understand. Hence, the MetFlex-Rx **Diet** prevailed.

Here is my issue with traditional diet books: For starters, most are incredibly ideological and dogmatic. As a whole, they leave little room for individuality within the diet. Just ask about eating the occasional vegetable in a Carnivore Diet forum or bananas in a Keto Diet Facebook group if you don't believe me. The Paleo, Keto, Plant-Based, and Carnivore Diet make bold, often unproven claims. Worse, if you question the claims made with genuine curiosity, you'll get roasted for it. You won't receive facts, direction, or meaningful debate—just anger. Diets put everyone in a 'box.' The apparent implication is that if you eat precisely the way the author or group suggests, you will succeed. When the diet doesn't work, it's because something is wrong with *you,* not with the way of eating.

The other common trend between diets is demonizing entire food groups. Every tribe needs a common enemy, and pointing out a high-level food group or macronutrient is the easiest way to label the opposition. If you read a keto book, fruit is a health concern. If you read a carnivore book, plants are poisonous. If you read a plant-based book, animal foods drive kidney disease and cancer. If all of these claims were accurate, what would be left to eat? It's not that traditional diets can't help some people. There are grains of truth to the underlying rules that a given diet espouses. But often, much-needed nuance is removed and replaced with strict dietary dogma.

For example, there are plant compounds that are problematic for a certain number of people. Look no further than peanuts. A single peanut can literally kill a significant number of humans on this planet. But those vulnerable people are the minority, not the majority. To look at the small population who suffers from peanuts and extrapolate the danger into population-wide mandates is silly. This is the kind of nonsense that is happening in carnivore communities, but not just with peanuts. Carnivore purists argue that all plants do more harm than good inside of the human body. The scale of extremity in this point of view varies from carnivore to carnivore.

Still, it remains a robust communal tone. Are you telling me that everyone in the world will get sick from eating blueberries and spaghetti squash? I doubt that.

You may be asking, 'but what about all the people who follow a given diet who become success stories?' The truth is that *any* structure is going to be beneficial for some percentage of the population. Also, when a person is most likely to seek out a new diet, she is probably at a nutritional low point in her life. When your diet consists of snacks, fast food, and alcohol, pretty much anything you do is going to give you excellent results. That is why small groups of people become so evangelistic about the diet they follow. When a way of eating makes a difference, you want to tell the world about it, and you genuinely want it to work for everyone you come in contact with. When a minority of loud, enthusiastic individuals begin to talk about a diet, it seems as though the entire planet is succeeding in their way of eating.

So what's the big deal if people want to scream the effectiveness of their diet from the rooftops? The issue is that dogmatic, restrictive, tribal diets don't work for most people in the long run. For the rare person, these diets can become a lifestyle. But most people require flexibility and a path to individualization to see long-term success. We are all different, and we need nuance in our dietary structure. The more restrictive or inflexible a person's diet, the more room to make 'mistakes.' The more 'mistakes' a person can make, the more opportunities he has to feel like a failure. Too many feelings of failure drive self-sabotage and self-sabotage is where progress ends. Diets that don't account for the flexibility necessary to manage the dieter's mindset fail most people.

The second part of the problem is the crucial variance between individuals not accounted for in diet tribes. The idea that all human beings should eat the same foods is quite frankly idiotic. People have different genetics, different ancestral origins, different dietary history, and different goals. These variables make cookie-cutter diets great for a few of us but problematic for most people. That is why I created the MetFlex-Rx approach. It is a dietary philosophy and structure that teaches the reader how to make food work for her—no hard rules. No dogma. Instead, a helpful path to give confidence and an amenable framework for the reader. The goal of the MetFlex-Rx diet is to have loose enough borders that the way of eating can evolve with the user.

If you are highly active and need to perform, more carbohydrates will likely be helpful for you. If you aren't very mobile and have a lot of weight to lose, starch and sugar are not your friends. The 36-year-old male CrossFitter and the 47-year-old female stay at home mother should not follow the same diet. These considerations must be made to make sense of the way you eat. When you follow the 'everyone should eat this, and not that' approach, individualization is lost, so are your results.

The Issue with Restriction Centric Diets

Successful diets must have some form of controlled consumption. People who say that you can eat as much as you want as long as it from a specific, limited group of food are bypassing standard science. I have heard industry ideologues say, "I have my clients eat 6000 calories per day, and as long as it's Keto, they lose weight". The idea that you can only gain weight by eating certain foods is ridiculous. You must reduce your total caloric intake, remove low-quality foods, or eat less frequently. Weight loss cannot exist without making some changes in these areas. People get into trouble by implemented dietary changes too quickly or in extreme ways.

Most of us want to lose weight, but being in a rush and taking large measures to reach our goals is often a mistake. Rapid weight loss can work for some people, but not for the vast majority of the population.

Restriction is followed by various psychological and physiological challenges. The faster the weight comes off of your body, the stronger your counter-regulatory weight loss system will push back. The result is often overconsumption and, sometimes, metabolic damage. The former makes losing weight more challenging now, and the latter hurts your chances of success in the future. Look at what happened to the biggest loser contestants. Most gained back excessive amounts of weight after their initial 'success' on the show. This rebound reaction is a common finding in weight loss literature. There are, of course, exceptions to this rule.

Sometimes a person loses a ton of weight and ends up keeping it off. You usually see this after health scares or other dramatic life changes (like the obese man who didn't eat for a year). However, smaller and more reasonable changes over time produce significant long-term results more frequently for the average person.

Summary

- A metabolically flexible person can metabolize both fat and carbohydrate. Depending on the day's energy demands, the flexible individual will shift back and forth between the two substrates.
- Fat is not bad for you- nor are carbohydrates.
- Protein is both safe and essential.

How you manage macronutrients as an individual makes the difference. The inappropriate consumption of any macronutrient can be a problem, but none are inherently unhealthy. Your body is designed to use protein, carbohydrates, and fats of all kinds when the individual need matches the intake. When your nutrient input is grossly mismatched with your level of activity, goals, and other lifestyle factors, you will gain weight and suffer. When you understand how to adjust what you eat to match your requirements, you lose fat, gain muscle, and thrive. This may sound complex on the surface, but the book aims to simplify these principles into straightforward and specific action steps. Let's get into it.

THE METFLEX-RX FUNDAMENTALS

In the fundamentals section of the book, I will cover a high-level overview of the diet. I intend to give you a clear understanding of why I recommend eating the way that I do. That way, once we get into the diet's details in the following section, you will know precisely why I structured things the way I did. So don't worry if you feel like you need greater detail while reading this chapter. The practical specifics of the diet will follow.

Whole Foods First

The majority of a successful person's progress comes from a few high-level actions, not the novel and exciting fads that come up on celebrity Instagram pages. The bland, obvious things we should do every day, are where the foundation for success is laid. Most people want to find the 'magic' that leads to great results. As a result, we get sucked into marketing for the latest fat-burning exercise trend or novel combinations of superfoods that promise to restore our youth. We seek out these hacks to save us from the simple, useful, daily tasks that lead to long-term results. In this section of the book, I want to layout the considerations that deliver 90% of your potential results.

The most critical action you can take to reach any goal is to eat primarily (if not exclusively) whole foods. This seems obvious, but many diets suggest tossing out entire food groups rather than including a diversity of high-quality foods.

Some people should eat a lot of meat, while others can be more plant dominant. Some people can thrive while including grains and dairy, while others should avoid them like the plague. Raw vegetables can be destructive for people with digestive issues. Simultaneously, those who have robust digestive systems can improve their gut biodiversity with fresh, raw produce.

There isn't a simple solution for everyone. But to decide you're going to eliminate fruit, meat, or vegetables just because some dweeb on Instagram convinced you to join his diet trend is senseless. Leave your options open at the high-level and don't jump right into dogmatic restrictions. There is always room to refine your diet, but your food philosophy should not begin with restriction. If you are maximizing whole foods and eliminating processed foods, you will get the vast majority of potential dietary results.

The more processed a food is, the more detrimental its consumption is for our well-being. This is true across the board. So what *is a* 'whole food'? In short, the closer to nature you can eat, the better. For starters, if it grows out of the ground or eats things that grow out of the earth, it is a whole food. Meat, vegetables, fruits, nuts, and seeds, and some grains and pseudo-grains would fall into this category.

Within the primary groups I mentioned, there are further layers of 'wholeness.' For instance, take an apple. Some people think apple juice is a whole food, but apple juice is hardly recognizable as an apple plucked from a tree. The amount of processing that happens after the apple is picked determines the food's 'wholeness.' An apple is more whole than apple sauce. Apple sauce is more whole than apple juice. Apple juice is more whole than a fruit rollup. Each stage of processing moves the food further away from its natural wholeness. With each step, the food becomes less beneficial. The further you move down the chain, the worse off you will be.

Rice is a staple of many Asian food cultures and can be a healthy part of many diets. But what about rice chips, rice crispies, or a chocolate cake which includes rice flour? You can get so far away from the original food that what you are eating doesn't even resemble what you are pretending to eat. So when I say 'whole foods' I mean as close to nature as possible. Some processing is O.K., but the closer you stay to the original product, the better your food choice will be.

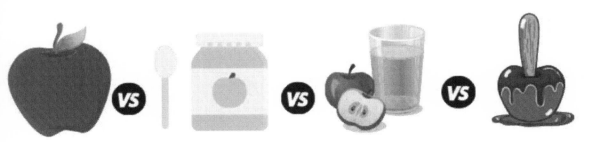

An apple, vs apple sauce, vs apple juice, vs a candied apple. The further you move from the original food and the more processing and additives that make their way into the final product, the worse off you will be.

Nutrient Density

Once you have taken a food's 'wholeness' into consideration, you should move to nutrient density. Nutrient density is the caloric cost you are paying for the amount of nutrition you are getting from any given food. Some foods are packed with vital nutrients and very little 'filler.' In contrast, other foods have *some.*

nutrients, but at the cost of significant filler and empty calories. Let's take high starch foods, for example. While rice can be an appropriate food to eat on occasion, that certainly doesn't make it ideal. The result of rice's high starch content is delivering lots of energy (calories) but minimal nutrition. It is essentially a filler food. Filler foods are great for survival when nutrient-dense foods are unavailable. But when you have the option to select something with fewer calories and greater nutritional value, rice becomes a poor choice. Starches might be useful for a high-level athlete who has great energy needs, but not for the average person who spends his day sitting at a desk.

Animal meats and above ground vegetables are examples of foods that deliver high nutritional value at a low caloric cost. In particular, animal foods are highly bioavailable, and the nutrients inside are easy for human beings to assimilate. Starchy foods like root vegetables and pseudo-grains (like quinoa) are not off-limits. Foods lower on the nutrient density pyramid just wouldn't be my top choice for most individuals. When you are looking to lose fat, gain muscle, and be energized, you want the maximum vitamins and minerals for the minimum caloric cost. That means that nutrient density matters and should play a role in your food selection.

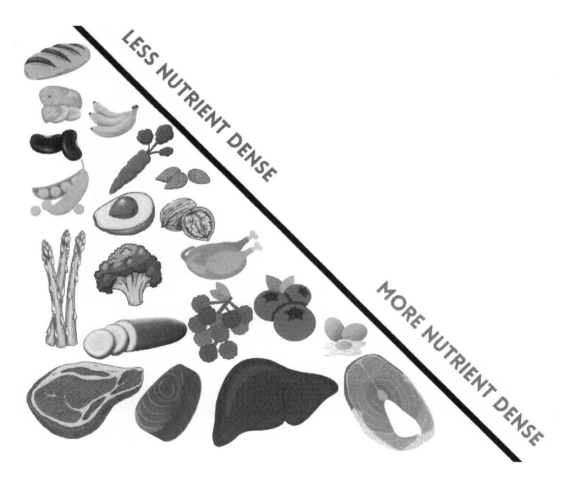

Protein Maximization

Many people are afraid to consume ideal amounts of protein. Studies suggest that protein from animal food is harmful are highly flawed, and the argument against protein is highly ideological. Most well-conducted research that has been done in the last decade shows the opposite. Protein appears to be at worst, neutral, and at best, essential for human health. As far as protein being a cause or driver of disease, this stance has been thoroughly debunked.

When it comes to something like fat loss, protein intake is critical. What is it that makes this macronutrient so essential to get right? For starters, protein is the most satiating macronutrient you can eat. High satiety makes protein almost impossible to overeat. Protein also has the highest thermic effect of all macronutrients. A high thermic effect means that you burn more calories digesting and metabolizing protein than you would when eating carbohydrates or fats. You can burn up to 30% of the protein calories you ingest by digestion alone. In my experience, the more protein a person eats at each meal, the better control that person has over other palatable foods.

Protein acts as a moderator for overeating and helps prevent the individual from overeating consequential foods. People who don't eat enough protein often struggle to regulate their diet and end up overeating both carbohydrates *and* fats. In fact, it is hypothesized that intense cravings for carbohydrates are driven by protein deficiency. However you look at it, protein matters, and if you aren't getting enough in your diet, you will suffer.

The Protein (to energy) Ratio

There is also the protein ratio to consider. This is a similar concept to nutrient density, only with protein as the anchor you want to maximize instead of vitamins and minerals. When it comes to weight loss, you want to eat foods that give you the most protein at the lowest caloric cost. You want to stick to leaner meats and other protein sources that carry less fat content- or in the case of dairy- fewer carbohydrates as well.

I want to be clear that I am not attempting to demonize fat by highlighting the protein ratio. Animal fat is not something to fear, and fattier cuts of meat are some of the most valuable, nutrient-dense foods on the planet. It is the highly refined seed oils that you should be avoiding. But when weight loss and fat loss are the goals, fattier cuts of meat can hinder your progress. For some, fatty foods are easy to over-consume, especially when you have issues with appetite control. If you carry a lot of body fat, chances are you have a problem with overconsumption.

I would not suggest focusing on leaner cuts of meat to a person with single-digit body fat, but chances are that isn't you. By nature of this being a fat loss book, I can assume that caloric control will be necessary for your success. Think about the protein ratio while selecting this vital nutrient.

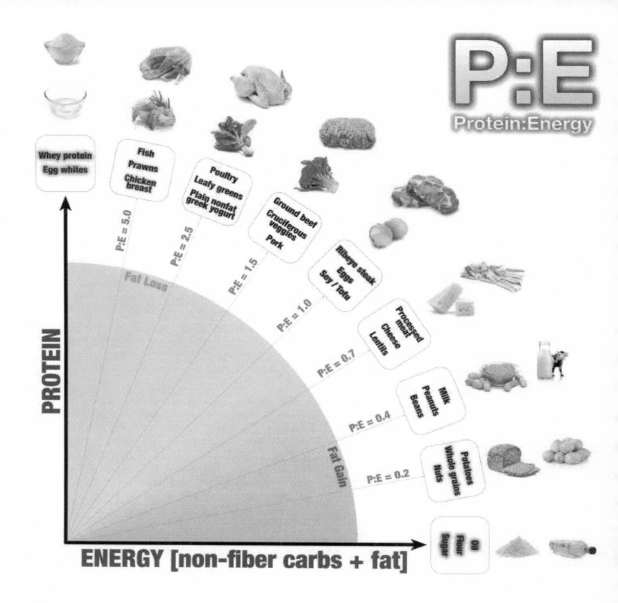

I took this image from Ted Naiman. He is a leader in this space. Check out his work if you want to learn more about P/E Ratios.

Carb Management

Carbohydrates get a bad rap. In most anti-carb circles, *all* carbohydrates get grouped together. A blueberry and a blueberry muffin are often indistinguishable from each other inside the silos of these diet tribes. Carbohydrates *can* be an issue for fat loss. Still, the type and quantity of the carbs you consume are highly variable. The right amount of the ideal type can be helpful in many ways. The wrong amount from poor sources will get you into trouble.

Problems result from consuming high amounts of carbohydrates while also being inactive, or when the carbohydrates we consume are highly refined or full of sugar. When you combine starch and sugar with a body that isn't in motion, you're going to have weight and fat gain. This is when 'carb matching becomes critical.' Carb matching is titrating your carbohydrate intake up or down to match your activity duration and intensity. Doing so can supplement your exercise performance and recovery without sacrificing your waistline. Sweet potatoes, strawberries, and even the occasional cup of rice are helpful foods for the high-intensity exerciser.

Starchy carbs can also be a useful psychological crutch when dieting. Consuming a planned amount of ideal carbohydrates can stop you from going overboard with foods you struggle with.

For the average person who sits for most of the day and exercises just a few times each week, starch and sugar, even from the healthiest sources, are fat loss barriers.

Carbs are fun to eat. Sweet and Starchy foods are also powerful forms of self-medication for stress, anxiety, and sadness. The comfort we get from carbs is what makes this food group so challenging to control. If you can manage your intake, you can continue to reap psychological rewards without hurting your physique. Just remember that I am referencing whole foods, not sports drinks and sugar packets. There are clearly carbohydrate-based junk foods that don't have a place in any person's diet. But there *is* a place in most people's diets for carbohydrates from whole food sources. Management is the key.

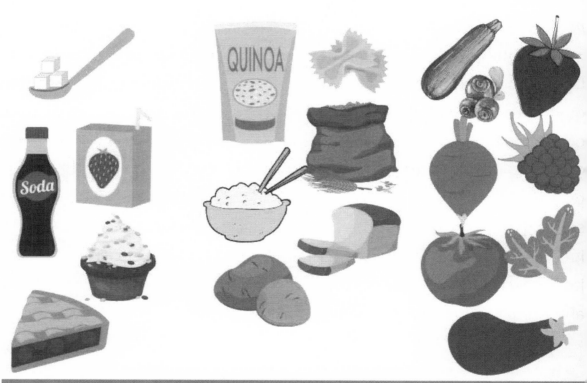

| Unhealthy | Unhealthy to Neutral | Neutral to Healthy |

All foods above are 'Carbs'

Fat is healthy, but not in excess

Much of the nutrition world has overcome the fear of fat that began with Ancel Keys and sugar industry lobbyists'. However, for those around in the '80s, the underlying fear of fat is still intense. Dietary fat is not just healthy to consume. It is essential for human health. Fatty fish, olive oil, nuts and seeds, and other whole food sources of fat are critical for the human body's proper function. Some people need more fat, and some people need less fat. Some people can thrive with significant saturated fat. Others will do better by replacing some saturated fat with monounsaturated fats instead. But everyone *needs* fat.

Like most foods, the quality of the fat you consume makes all the difference. When fat comes from processed food, seed oils, shortening, and other trans fats, it becomes a health issue. When combined in high quantities with processed sugar (like in most packaged foods), fat is a problem. But when consumed in moderate amounts from whole food sources, fat can be powerful health food. We will get into the details of fat intake and ideal sources once we get to how to structure your diet. For now, just know that not all fats are created equal, and knowing which to consume and which to avoid is the most critical consideration.

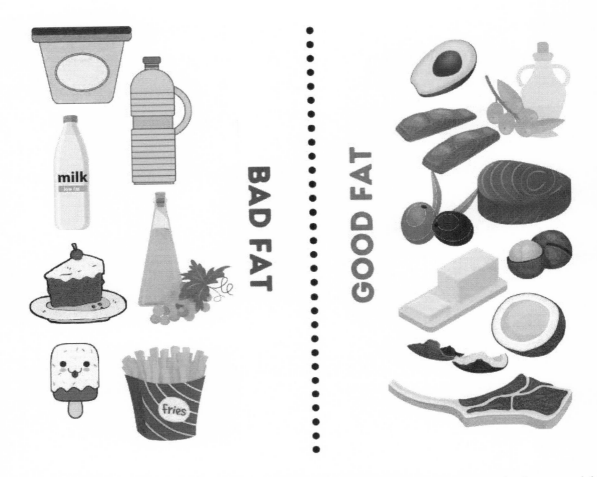

Good Fats: Naturally occurring fats with little processing (aside from cold pressing or mixing)

Bad Fats: Hydrogenated and highly refined oils found in most seed oils, baking, frying, and processed foods.

This concludes the high-level overview of the MetFlex-Rx Fundamentals. Now we can move onto the diet's details and how you can apply them to your current fitness strategy.

THE DETAILS OF THE DIET

In this section of the book, we will begin building your diet. It all starts with food selection. The primary food groups in the MetFlex-Rx diet are proteins, healthy fats, high starch carbohydrates, and low starch carbohydrates. This is the language we will use to understand how to categorize our foods and build our meals and snacks. Although I have already introduced you to the basic theory of our main macronutrients (proteins, carbs, and fats), we revisit them next in greater specificity.

Nutrient Classifications

Proteins:

animal proteins are preferred on this diet. When compared to plant proteins, they are more nutrient-dense and come with a lower caloric cost. That isn't to say that beans, legumes, nuts, seeds, and grains can't replace animal foods in your diet, but those foods are carbohydrate or fat-dominant foods with a little bit of protein inside. Many believe that nuts or beans are high protein foods. If you look at the non-protein caloric cost you're paying to get a small amount of protein from such foods, the assumption is not accurate. What we are looking for in this diet are protein-dominant foods. If you are vegetarian, you can still rely on eggs and high protein dairy, which will be helpful.

If you are 100% plant-based, you'll want to supplement your diet with high-quality protein powders that have had the starch removed. Brown rice protein, pea protein, and other options should help you hit your protein goals without overconsumption of starch and sugar. The main foods you will find in the protein category are red meat, chicken, pork, wild game, fish and seafood, organ meats, eggs, and high protein dairy.

The Protein Pyramid

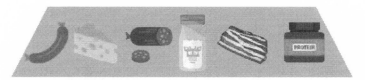

EAT SPARINGLY (A FEW TIMES PER WEEK)

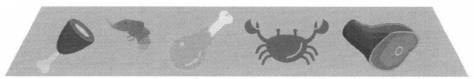

EAT OCCASIONALLY (UP TO ONCE PER DAY)

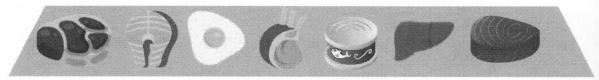

EAT ABUNDANTLY (UNLIMITED)

Abundantly: Ruminants (beef, lamb, game), fish (salmon, mackerel, tuna, cod), canned fish (tuna/salmon), whole eggs (if tolerant), organ meat (if accustomed)

Occasionally: Non-Ruminants (chicken, turkey, pork), crustaceans and shellfish (shrimp, crab, oysters, mussels)

Sparingly: Cured and processed meats, cheese, milk and milk based protein, protein powders and other protein supplements

Healthy Fats: healthy fats can come from both plants and animals. Unhealthy fats can come from both as well. Highly refined seed oils and processed animal fats are both a concern for your health. So do your best to stick to the fat source examples laid out in this list.

The Fat Pyramid

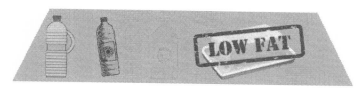

AVOID

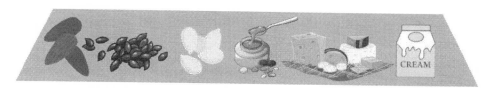

EAT ONCE PER DAY OR LESS

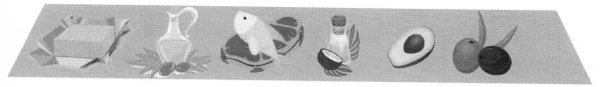

EAT AT EACH MEAL

Abundantly: Natural saturated and monounsaturated fats (butter, olive oil, macadamia nut oil, coconut oil), olives, avocado, and intrinsic fat in fatty meats

Occasionally: Nuts, seeds, nut/seed butter, cheese, and cream

Avoid: Refined seed oils (canola, peanut, sunflower etc.), trans fats, margarine and other low fat processed foods

Polyunsaturated and saturated fats can be controversial. Saturated fat because of its connection to cholesterol levels, and polyunsaturated fat due to its lack of stability and potential to drive oxidative damage. The great fat debate is a complex topic that I am not going to cover in this book. If you are getting your fat from unrefined, whole food sources, you shouldn't concern yourself with the finer details. Make monounsaturated fats the focus of your overall intake, followed by saturated fat. Polyunsaturated sources can make up the balance. Olive oil, fatty fish, macadamia nuts, and avocados are examples of foods that are high in monounsaturated fats. Most ruminant meat (beef, lamb, game) is about a 50/50 split of saturated to monounsaturated fat.

Low Starch Carbs: Low starch carbs come in the form of above-ground vegetables and berries from the fruit family. These are the carbohydrates that are going to deliver the most nutrition at the lowest caloric cost. Broccoli, brussels sprouts, kale, mushrooms, bok choy, blueberries, and raspberries are examples of low starch carbs.

High Starch Carbs: High starch carbs are whole plant foods that can be eaten on occasion but give less nutritional value at a higher caloric cost. Root vegetables, most fruits, grains and pseudo-grains fall into this category. Carrots, sweet potatoes, rice, quinoa, watermelon, and apples are the kinds of foods that carry the 'HSC' label. These foods are not 'unhealthy' but can be problematic when we mismanage them- which we often do.

High starch carbs are also the whole foods that we typically get the greatest psychological satisfaction from, making them easy to overeat. It can help keep high starch carbohydrates in your diet for psychological relief and food satisfaction. But only if you're reasonably active and capable of keeping your intake under control.

The Carbohydrate Pyramid

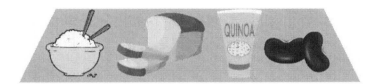

EAT SPARINGLY (WHEN INTENSELY ACTIVE)

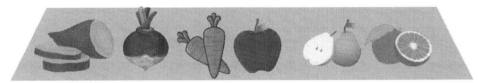

EAT OCCASIONALLY (ON ACTIVE DAYS)

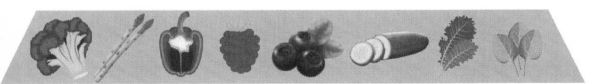

EAT ABUNDANTLY (UNLIMITED)

Abundantly: Above ground vegetables and berries from the fruit family

Only on active days: Roots, tubers, and the rest of the fruit family

Only on intensely active days and if clearly tolerable: Rice, wheat, beans and pseudo-grains

Meal Frequency

Meal frequency is simply the number of times you eat over the day. How many meals and snacks you have and the amount of time you go between eating play a role in the frequency equation.

If you are just beginning your transformation, it may be best to start with three meals per day or three meals per day with one or two snacks. The only purpose of snacking is to have planned psychological food breaks to prevent binge eating more consequential foods. Eventually, it would be best to ween yourself down to less frequent eating and removing snacking. Most people will see the best results with two meals per day or two meals plus a snack. The popularized idea that eating frequently leads to increased metabolism and greater fat burning is inaccurate.

Constant consumption of food pushes up your blood sugar and insulin levels and minimizes your opportunity for fat loss. When you eat, your blood sugar rises. When your blood sugar elevates, you produce the hormone insulin to move the blood sugar out of the bloodstream and into various tissues. While insulin is being made, glucose is prioritized for energy use, and fat burning is virtually shut off. The more frequently you eat, the more often you turn on this process, and the less regularly you access stored fat.

The adipose tissue found on your body that you are trying to rid of is your 'last resort' for energy needs. When you have other energy substrates to use like alcohol, glucose, or circulating fatty acids from a recent meal, you are not going to effectively dip into your fat stores.

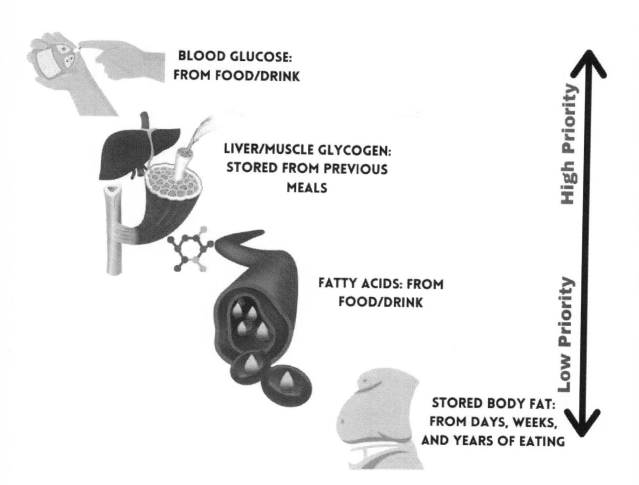

BLOOD GLUCOSE: FROM FOOD/DRINK

LIVER/MUSCLE GLYCOGEN: STORED FROM PREVIOUS MEALS

FATTY ACIDS: FROM FOOD/DRINK

STORED BODY FAT: FROM DAYS, WEEKS, AND YEARS OF EATING

High Priority

Low Priority

Setting Up Main Meals

Most people should aim to eat 2-3 meals per day. The more space you can have between meals, the better. I make this suggestion because when you're eating, you're not burning fat. In short, when you eat, your blood sugar rises. When blood sugar rises, you produce the hormone insulin, which shuttles glucose from the bloodstream and around the body. When this process is on, fat burning is off. Using stored fat for energy is low on the fuel priority list. If you have alcohol, fatty acids, or high glucose levels in the blood, fat won't be burned efficiently. The easiest way to change this dynamic is to go time without food.

The old maxim that you should eat many small meals frequently throughout the day to stoke your metabolism is false. Extending time between meals gives your body the chance to use its own excess calories, thus, increasing fat loss potential.

In a few pages you'll see where I have broken down meals and serving sizes for both men and women into two to three meals per day. First, I want to go over some serving size and hand measurement details.

Serving Sizes

Servings sizes aren't a science, and you don't need to obsess over them. But it is helpful to begin your diet with some method of control. I like to use a basic hand measurement system to give people an idea of what a 'serving' looks like without getting obsessive. In this system, a serving of protein is the size of your palm, a serving of low starch carbohydrates is the size of your fist, a serving of high starch carbohydrates is the size of what you could fit in your palm, and a serving of fat is the size of your thumb. These are ballpark measurements, and as long as you are attempting to integrate some sort of food intake control, you'll get the benefit.

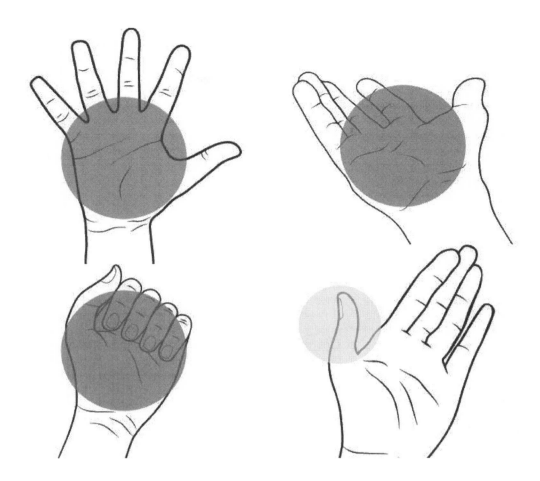

Men: 3 Meals (servings listed are per meal)

1-2 servings of protein

1-2 servings of fat

1-2 serving of low starch carbs

1 TOTAL serving of high starch carbs (one per day in only one meal)

Men: 2 Meals (servings listed are per meal)

2-3 servings of protein

2-3 servings of fat

1-2 servings of low starch carbs

1 TOTAL serving of high starch carbs (one per day in only one meal)

Men: 3 Meals

1-2 servings of protein
1-2 servings of fat
1-2 serving of low starch carbs
1 TOTAL serving of high starch carbs
(one per day in only one meal)

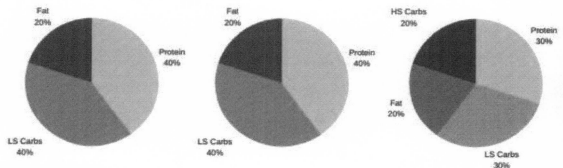

Men: 2 Meals

2-3 servings of protein
2-3 servings of fat
2-3 servings of low starch carbs
1 TOTAL serving of high starch carbs
(one per day in only one meal)

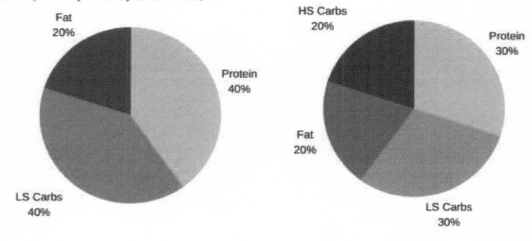

Women: 3 Meals (servings shown are per meal)

1-2 servings of protein

1 serving of fat

1-2 servings of low starch carbs

1 serving of high starch carbs TOTAL (one serving in one meal. Not in all feeds)

Women: 2 Meals (servings shown are per meal)

2-3 servings of protein

2 servings of fat

1-3 servings of low starch carbs

1 serving of high starch carbs TOTAL (one serving in one meal. Not in all feeds)

Women: 3 Meals

1-2 servings of protein
1 serving of fat
1-2 servings of low starch carbs
1 serving of high starch carbs TOTAL
(one serving in one meal. Not in all
feeds)

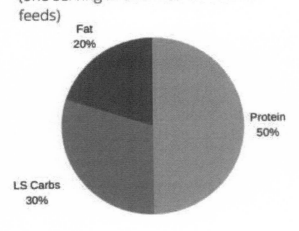

Women: 2 Meals

2-3 servings of protein
2 servings of fat
1-3 servings of low starch carbs
1 serving of high starch carbs TOTAL
(one serving in one meal. Not in all
feeds)

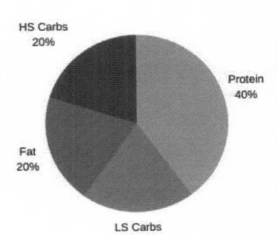

As a reminder, below are the types of foods you should aim to fill your meals with. Simply combine your hand measurement system with your four basic categories of food while using the meal composition template examples above. Nutrition does not need to be more complicated than that.

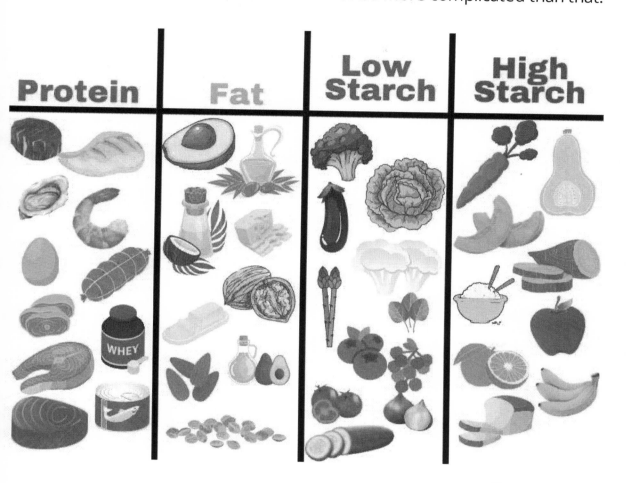

When to add high starch carbs

High starch carbohydrates should be reserved for days when you have higher energy demands. The higher the intensity and the longer the duration of your exercise or sport, the more high starch carbohydrates you can eat. You also need to consider your weight and fat loss goals when considering your starch intake. The more weight you have to lose and the greater the importance you place on fat loss- the less starchy carbs you should eat- regardless of your activity level. So essentially, you have three factors to consider when deciding how many starchy carbs you'll consume on a day to day basis.

1. How active you are
2. How much of a priority weight loss and fat loss is to you
3. How much psychological satisfaction you need from healthy comfort food to keep you away from junk food

All three of these factors are legitimate reasons to increase or decrease your starchy carb intake.

Determining a Baseline

If you are inactive and sitting at a desk for most of the day, your baseline high starchy carb intake should be 0-1 servings. What determines whether you start with 0 or 1 are factors two and three from the previous list. If fat loss is critically important to you, start with 1 serving. If not having any starchy carbohydrates in your baseline diet will drive you nuts, add one in. Focus on more important factors like the consistency of exercise and whole foods consumption.

The more you exercise and the higher your exercise's intensity, the more starchy foods you can consume. Again, the more fat loss matters to you, the less true this is. Perhaps it's better stated that the more intensely active you are, the more starchy carbs you can get away with eating. In any case, you can consider adding a maximum of one serving of high starch carbs for each of the activities below.

45 minutes of weightlifting

20-30 minutes of HIIT training

60 minutes of sport

45 minutes of swimming

60 minutes of moderately difficult yoga

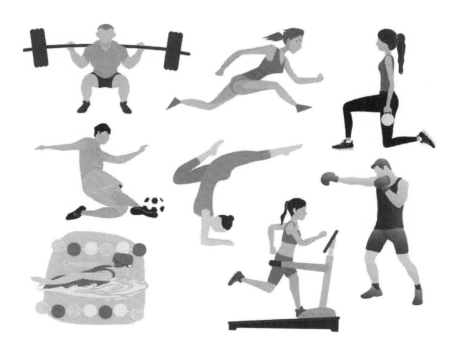

These are just a few examples. The general rule is that if your exercise causes burning muscles, burning lungs, or profuse sweating- and goes on for at least 30 minutes- you can add a carb serving to your baseline. If not, your exercise does not allow for additional carbs. Without any intense exercise carbs don't have a dietary purpose. If you have a single bout of intense exercise, you can consider supplementing with a single starchy carbohydrate serving. If you have multiple intense bouts of exercise, you could justify consuming multiple starchy carb sources (if performance and recovery align with your goals).

InActive Day

Active Day

Intensely Active Day

Remember, you don't *have* to increase your starch intake on days when you are more active. Your fat loss is going to be greater if you keep your starchy carb intake down. But if you are going to increase your starchy carb intake, this is the time to do it. You need to earn it.

Fat Burning Exercises

Activities of lower intensity and longer duration like walking, light jogging, stretching, etc. are primarily fat burning exercises. This doesn't mean that you couldn't add some high starch carbs on days when you perform them; it just won't help with weight loss and fat loss. Lower intensity 'fat-burning' activities don't require carbohydrates to be adequately performed. The higher and faster the energy demand, the more glucose is needed and used by the body. The lower and slower the demand for energy, the more fat used (in relative terms). An all-out sprint uses the most glucose, while sleeping is predominantly a fat-burning activity.

To be clear, this doesn't mean you burn more fat in an hour of sleeping than in an hour of wind sprints. It just means that the relative ratio of fat burned (comparative to carbohydrates) is higher. The total energy used in the activity will determine the higher total amount of fat loss. So if you are active but less intensely, you should be minimizing your high starchy carbohydrate intake. If you are active and very intense, a higher starchy carb intake will help your performance.

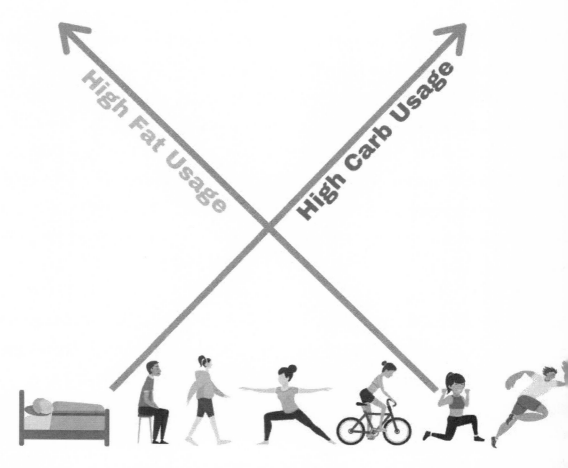

The lower the intensity and energy demand, the more fat we use. The greater the intensity and energy demand, the more we rely on carbohydrates. This is not to say that the human body can't adapt to perform higher intensity exercise on a low carb diet. It is, however, much more likely that performance will suffer on the high intensity end without carb supplementation.

It is really that simple. Eat those foods, in those quantities, with a controlled meal frequency, and you'll move the needle on your progress.

What About My Snacks?

As I briefly mentioned, the less snacking you do, the better. But if you know that grazing and frequent eating is an area you struggle with, it is better to be well-prepared. Instead of believing you will access willpower and avoid convenient, unhealthy foods, I'd prefer you to make some readily available snacks from the list below. Just remember that snacking is psychologically driven. It isn't a matter of hunger. It is a matter of stimulation or using food as an escape or a stimulus. There is an opportunity to snack healthily as long as you pre-make healthy replacements for the craving mechanism you have.

Suppose you have not already prepared a healthy snack when a psychological craving comes. In that case, you will default to an unhealthy option. So have at least 2-3 snacks premade every day- just in case.

You are going to snack, and you are going to indulge. You will turn to food when you are stressed, tired, sad, mad, and bored. You will have moments of weakness. So you'd best be prepared.

Eating food to stimulate or escape emotional turmoil is better than drinking two bottles of wine or punching someone in the throat, so give yourself some leeway. In these moments, you will go for the most convenient food that fits your functional snacking mechanism. Some of us like to crunch, others need sweetness and texture, and some need richness and volume. We usually fill these cravings with stuff like chips, ice cream, and pizza. Hunger and cravings quickly become an emergency that we extinguish with the most problematic foods.

You'd be surprised by how satisfying healthy options can be in thes[e] scenarios as long as the healthy choice is *as convenient* as the unhealth[y] option. Dehydrated zucchini chips can be as gratifying as regular chips. Som[e] almonds, cashews, and mixed berries can be as satisfying as a chocolate bar. Some powdered peanut butter, raw cacao, and greek yogurt can be a[s] enjoyable as ice cream. The catch is that healthy options take effort t[o] make. When an emotional craving comes, you don't have time to cu[t,] dehydrate, and mix healthy replacement options. This is where preparatio[n] is paramount. If you have healthy snack replacements ready to go in a tim[e] of need, you will eat them first, and you'll feel a lot better about it.

First, you need to establish which of the following you are: a cruncher, [a] sweet-tooth, or a richness eater.

CRUNCHER

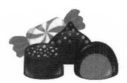 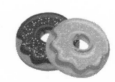 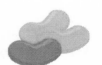

SWEET-TOOTH

 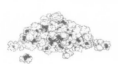 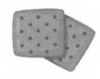 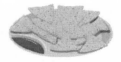

RICHNESS/FULLNESS

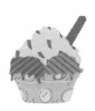 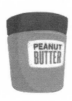 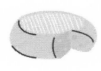

You could have one, or you could have all of these craving mechanisms. Once you identify your craving type, start making batches of healthy alternatives for your moments of weakness. Crunchers need stuff like kale chips, zucchini chips, root vegetable chips, and even commercially bought veggie straws can be O.K. on occasion. Sweet tooths often need texture and sweetness in combination. This can almost always be achieved with mixed nuts and mixed berries: blueberries and almonds, cashews and raspberries, macadamia, and strawberries will all suffice. Aim to use more berries than nuts at a 4:1 ratio. You can even mix some high cacao dark chocolate cubes if you need to. All combinations will work, and the goal is to move away from the destructive foods you usually succumb to.

Richness eaters can satisfy cravings with greek yogurt, skyr, or labneh mixed with powdered peanut butter or your favorite protein powder. Some richness eaters can also make snack loaves with eggs, zucchini, chia seeds, and other high fiber foods.

CRUNCHER

- DEHYDRATED KALE CHIPS
- DEHYDRATED ZUCCHINI CHIPS
- SPIRALIZED BAKED AND SALTED VEGETABLES
- VEGGIE STRAWS

SWEET-TOOTH

- MIXED BERRIES WITH NUTS/SEEDS AND DARK CACAO CHOCOLATE
- SMOOTHIE WITH YOUR FAVOURITE FRUITS, A BIT OF DAIRY AND PROTEIN POWDER

RICHNESS/FULLNESS

- PANCAKE WITH 5 EGGS, 1/4 TBSP OF GROUND OATMEAL, TOPPED WITH SWEET AVOCADO MOUSSE
- GREEK YOGURT, PROTEIN POWDER, AND POWDERED PEANUT BUTTER MIX

Get creative with it. Just know that when the craving comes, you will no whip something up quickly, so don't make the mistake of not having you snack replacement on hand. If you are unprepared, you're going to tea open a bag of chips that you will regret eating. So have at least 2-3 option readily available every night (or whenever snack cravings are the stronges for you).

Lastly, if it's in your budget, some helpful technologies make healthy snack creation a cinch. Below I have listed my favorite tools for cutting, chopping mixing, and drying my snacks.

Immersion Blender: use to create a whipped texture for rich foods like avocado, greek yogurt, and other fatty food replacements.

Food Processor: use to thinly slice foods you want to dehydrate or grind foods you want to add to healthy pancakes or muffins.

Dehydrator: you can get a decent dehydrator for less than $100. This tool is essential if you struggle with crunchy, snacky foods. Kale chips, zucchin chips, and your own dried berries can be made for your snack mix.

Mandolin: If thin-slicing is all you need for your snacks and you don't want to invest in a food processor, and mandolin will do the trick for $30

Spiralizer: use to turn squash, zucchini, carrots, and other firm vegetables into noodles you can use to accompany your favourite dinner dishes

How to Adjust Your Template When Progress Stalls

The instructions on meal frequency, serving sizes, and snacking are a general template. Different people are going to need to make various changes along the way. One way to customize your diet is to adjust your carbohydrate intake to match your goal and level of activity. The second way of managing your dietary intake is to reduce (or increase) servings on a scale based on what is or is not happening in terms of your progress.

You must give your diet at least 2-4 weeks of consistency at a time before you make any adjustments to your overall food intake. If you are three days in and your scale goes up a pound, please resist the urge to rush to make changes. Reductions in caloric intake can be helpful, but there is only so much runway you have with caloric interventions- and if you rush to reduce the amount of food you are eating in the hopes of losing more weight quickly, your plan will backfire.

So assuming you have given your current template at least two weeks, and you have not seen any weight/fat loss or, worse, weight/fat gain, this is how you can scale your adjustments.

Step 1- Reduce Your Starchy Carb Intake: Assuming you have been having 1-3 servings of starchy carbs per day, bring those down one at a time. If you are having three, reduce them to two per day. If you are having two, reduce them to one per day. Don't bring down your starchy carb intake by more than one serving at a time, and don't make any reductions without a two-week buffer in between. If, after two weeks, the scale begins to move, do not push further decreases.

Step 2- Reduce Your Fat Intake: Assuming you are having more than three servings of fat per day, you can reduce your fat (one serving at a time) down to a minimum of three fat servings per day. There should not be any reason to go below one serving of fat per meal. The same rules apply for fat reductions as carb reductions; you should only drop one serving at a time and never more within two weeks. If, after two weeks, the scale moves, don't reduce any further. If you are currently eating many fatty cuts of meat, you can also move to leaner sources of protein.

You should never go below three servings of protein, three servings of healthy fat, and 3-5 servings of low starch carbohydrates in a day. If this is currently the amount of food you are consuming, and you still are not losing body fat, you need to:

A- focus on increasing your level of activity, your amount of quality sleep, reducing stress, and considering other lifestyle functions

or

B- See a professional. You may have some significant hormonal (or other) health issues going on that require a medical professional. A is much more likely than B, but B is still possible and a scenario to consider.

STRATEGIES AND TACTICS

Before I get into strategies that can help maximize your results, let me say this: **90% of the progress you make will come from what you eat and how you move your body**. Applying what you have learned in the sections leading up to this point will be far more valuable than anything you will learn from this point on. Don't get caught in the trap of looking for strategies to save you from lacking efforts in diet and exercise. If you are not giving diet and exercise your full commitment, steps in this process will not lead to success. If you are already doing the necessary nutrition and exercise work, these tacts can maximize your results.

Time-Restricted Eating

TRE is a straightforward way that you can spend more time burning fat and becoming insulin sensitive. As I mentioned earlier, more frequent eating is not beneficial. Most people would be better off with a shorter eating window. TRE provides a strict start and stop time for eating. And for many people, a black and white cut off is easy to manage.

Most people should begin with a 12-hour fasting window, and most active people don't need to go beyond 16 hours of time restriction. That means that if you had your last meal at 8 PM the night before, you should not eat the next day until between 8 AM and 12 PM the following day. Essentially, you are pushing back breakfast or skipping it altogether. 'Skip breakfast,' you say, 'but that's the most important meal of the day!' The only people pushing breakfast as the most important meal of the day are cereal and bacon manufacturers.

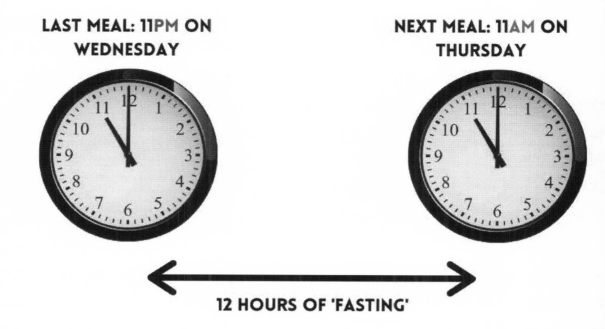

LAST MEAL: 11PM ON WEDNESDAY

NEXT MEAL: 11AM ON THURSDAY

12 HOURS OF 'FASTING'

Know Yourself, and Don't Bite Off More than You Can Chew

If you are currently a frequent eater, don't make the mistake of pushing long eating restriction windows. If you do, you will suffer and get little benefit from time-restricted eating. Begin with the 12-hour window. Give it two weeks, see how it goes. If you feel great, both physically and psychologically, go up to 14 hours. Give it two more weeks, see how you feel, and then consider going up to 16 hours. If, at any point, you get heavy brain fog, fatigue, headaches, or any adverse side effects during the fasting window, you may be doing too much too quickly. Back off to a window that is psychologically challenging but does not cause you physical suffering. Don't be in a rush to get results. You can get there without gritting your teeth if you listen to your body.

Occasional Intermittent Fasting

Time-restricted eating and intermittent fasting are often used interchangeably. The intermittent fasting label should be reserved for extended periods of fasting. TRE is simply a controlled eating window. In this example of intermittent fasting, I am referring to 24-hour fasts.

Occasional, prolonged fasting can help increase your insulin sensitivity and glucose control. I also find it is incredibly helpful for improving psychological resilience and reducing problematic cravings. You 'toughen up' the mind when you refuse any and all cravings for an extended period. Some people intermittent fast to increase 'autophagy'- the process of cellular clean-up, but this can be accomplished by much simpler means (like exercise). The data on this complex process is limited, so I am hesitant to suggest that fasting will increase your health at the cellular level.

I prefer time-restricted eating for my regular practice and perform intermittent fasts only on occasion. Once per month at most, and once per quarter at minimum.

Intermittent fasting isn't for everyone, but some people actually prefer it to TRE. An example of a 24 hour fast would be if you stopped eating at 8 PM on Tuesday night, you wouldn't eat again until between 8 PM and 9 PM on Wednesday. It's just as simple as counting 24 hours from your last meal. I would not suggest trying a 24 hour fast before practicing time-restricted eating first. TRE is more manageable, so see how you fare with it first. I also suggest that you try intermittent fasting when you are busy and productive. Otherwise, you'll be sitting around and thinking about food, and it'll be a miserable experience. If you decide to give fasting a try, start with one fast per month of a maximum of 24-36 hours.

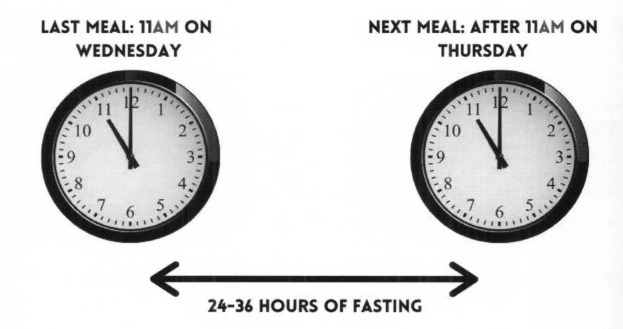

LAST MEAL: 11AM ON WEDNESDAY

NEXT MEAL: AFTER 11AM ON THURSDAY

24-36 HOURS OF FASTING

*Note- if you have ever experienced disordered eating, both binges *and* purges, fasting is not a practice you should take on. It can quickly become a problematic obsession for those demographics. There are many other ways to reach your goal without the associated risk.

Fasted Low-Intensity Exercise

Another way that we can achieve significant fat-burning is with fasted exercise. We force the adaptation to use fat more effectively when energy is in high demand, and body fat is our only fuel source. This is also a practice I do daily. I find that I am leaner because of it, but my workouts are actually more effective on an empty stomach. I'm not saying that will be your experience, and feeling good with fasted exercise takes time. If you try to exercise intensely on an empty stomach, you'll likely regret it. I am just sharing my personal practice. For most people, fasted low-intensity exercise is both simple and effective.

Walking, stretching, yoga, and light jogging can be done in the absence of food quite comfortably. Low intensity fasted training allows you to get the reward of the adaptation without the misery of performing intense exercise without adequate fuel. So don't get crazy with it and stick to the basics. Walking on an empty stomach in the morning is where everyone should begin.

The No, Low, Slow Carb Protocol

If fasting and time-restricted eating don't sound like your cup of tea, you can implement the No, Low, Slow Carb Method. I created this approach so people could become metabolically flexible without having to fast or restrict themselves. Especially if you're just starting out, this may be a better option for you. The 'NLSC' approach is accomplished by intelligently organizing your daily carbohydrate intake to delay the amount of sugar that ends up in your bloodstream after meals. Doing so can increase your ability to burn fat. This could be described as a sort of 'fast mimicking diet.' Below is an example of no, low, slow-carb eating.

If you are a three meal per day eater, you would have:

- 0-5 grams of carbohydrates in your first meal
- less than 15 grams carbohydrates only from above ground vegetables in your second meal
- and a single serving of complex carbohydrates (around 30 grams) in your last meal

This formula keeps your blood sugar and insulin levels down for as long as possible, even while eating, to encourage higher fat utilization. Here is an example of what a day of no, low, and slow carb eating would look like:

Here are some example meals that fit this formula

Meal #1 (No Carb) 4 whole eggs, a 1/4 cup of nuts, and some bone broth

Meal #2 (Low Carb) Greens salad with chicken breast and an oil and vinegar dressing

Meal #3 (Slow Carb) 8 oz Flank Steak with a side salad and 1/2 a sweet potato or 3/4 cup of cooked rice

or

First Meal: (No Carb) Two whole hard-boiled eggs, tuna, avocado

Second meal: (Low Carb) Spinach and kale salad with olive oil, sea salt, and one full can of Tuna

Third meal: (Slow Carb) Ground turkey with mixed vegetables on brown rice with ½ sweet potato

MEAL #1 MEAL #2 MEAL #3

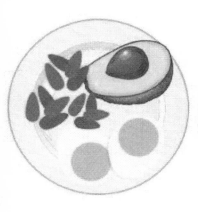 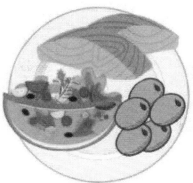 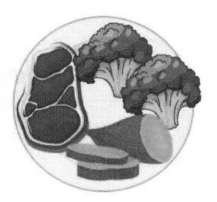

Below is an example food list in each meal category that you can use to reference what foods to eat and when while on the no, low, slow carb process.

No Carb Meals: Fish, fowl, beef, chicken, shrimp, crab, some nuts and seeds, avocado, eggs, egg whites, smoked meats, olive oil, coconut oil, avocado oil and spices, seasonings, sea salt.

Low Carb Meals: Add spinach, kale, chard, collards, broccoli, cabbage, peppers, zucchini, mushrooms, cauliflower, green beans, lettuce, brussels sprouts, celery, artichokes.

Slow Carb Meals: Add sweet potato, yams, lentils, brown rice, lima beans, split green peas, and steel-cut oats. Keep the serving size to roughly the size of your palm or less.

You can get lost in the specifics when it comes to carbohydrate measurements, but just remember that if you follow the basics, you'll get 90% of the results. So in meal one, stick to meat and fats. In meal two, add in some above-ground vegetables. In meal three, include a starchy carbohydrate source. If you do that, you'll be fine. Measuring carbs to the gram is unnecessary.

This concludes the section on strategies and tactics. If you have already proven your ability to stick to the diet basics, you should pick the one (and only one) method that you believe will fit best into your lifestyle. So try time restricted eating, intermittent fasting, or the low, no slow-carb protocol. Do not try to do them all at once. You will fall flat on your face.

BEHAVIOUR CHANGE

The last but most important aspect of nutrition you need to consider when setting a goal is behavior change. Behavior change is a tactic for overcoming the underlying driving forces of harmful choice-making. You may be wondering why choice-making matters more than what foods you do or don't eat. Let me address your skepticism with a few questions of my own.

What prevents you from doing what you already know you should do more of, like eating whole foods and exercising? Why can't you stop doing what you know you need to do less of, like eating junk food and watching three hours of youtube every night? The obsession with diet and exercise solutions while ignoring core behavioral problems is the average person's fitness dilemma. If you don't address your destructive eating behaviors, no broad nutritional strategy will help you. Overeating, late-night snacking, constant grazing, and binge eating are just a few of the average person's negative habits.

My first book, Heavy Brain, detailed the causes and solutions to these behavioral issues. If you struggle with unhealthy food behaviors, I suggest you read it. In the meantime, I have provided some easy tips you can follow right now to begin managing your relationship with food.

Eat Sitting Down

This seems simple enough, but how often do you eat sitting down at a table without distraction? We eat at our desks, in front of the T.V., and while staring at our smartphones. Heck, some of us eat in our beds! The issue with distracted eating is that it disconnects us from the food experience we are supposed to be having. If you are distracted while eating, you will ignore clear satiety signals, and thus, you are more likely to overeat. Secondly, we all require a certain amount of satisfaction from our food before being psychologically fulfilled. The more distracted you are while you eat, the less of a satisfying experience you will have. When psychologically unsatisfied we eat more.

We consume to make up for lack of eating fulfillment. So eat sitting down rid yourself of distractions, and chew slowly. You'll be amazed by how well this helps control your overeating.

Take 5 Minutes with the First Five Bites

To create a better connection and greater satisfaction with your food, you should spend 3-5 minutes chewing the first five bites. It doesn't matter if it is a snack or a meal; the rule still applies. It is challenging to eat mindlessly when you are spending 30-60 seconds chewing a mouthful of food, and avoiding mindless eating is key to the prevention of overconsumption. When we take our time with the first few bites and ask subtle questions about the taste, texture, and experience of the food, it sets the mind for a relaxed eating experience. This tactic will deliver the same satisfaction and control as eating sitting down. Try it; it works!

Be Productive at Night

When the end of the day comes, we typically become idle and unproductive. When we become unproductive, problematic emotions rise to the surface. We get bored, sad, anxious, or stressed. Once overwhelmed by these emotions, we do whatever it takes to rid of them. Food, alcohol, and technological distraction are the most effective ways to soothe ourselves while wrestling with emotional turmoil. This form of self-medication is a core reason why food habits are hard to break. I call the craving and consumption driving by a lack of productivity the 'downtime dilemma.' Everything from boredom to deep sadness comes up when we are in our most unfruitful states, and when this happens, we eat.

We eat to numb, stimulate, and distract ourselves from the distress. One solution to this potential issue is to sit with our emotions and face them head-on rather than escape the discomfort. Over time you learn to accept the ebb and flow of our various psychological states. When you no longer need to run from your inner monologue, you no longer need to medicate your mind with food, alcohol, and technological distraction. Working through emotional sensitivities can be a long road for most people (see Heavy Brain), so in the meantime, productivity can become a useful crutch.

If, instead of hitting the couch and becoming idle, you went for a short walk, read a book, or did some yoga, you could avoid succumbing to food as medicine. I call this method of changing your downtime habits 'shaking up the circuitry'.

When you intentionally schedule meaningful activity into the spaces where you are usually sluggish, you change the brain's pattern that typically results in destructive eating. In the past, you have programmed yourself to be lazy and distracted in your downtime. When you are idle and mindless, your brain has been instructed to ask for food. This is the wiring that you have reinforced over the past several years. If you schedule a productive activity when you are usually sitting on the couch or staring at your smartphone, your mind stops asking for food-based distractions. This intervention won't change your cravings immediately.

Still, over time, you will literally rewire your brain away from poor eating habits. When you are at your least active, try an engaging activity of mind, body, or both. You will see the difference it can make when it comes to problematic eating behaviors. The downtime dilemma is most common between dinner and bedtime. Depending on your schedule, this could be different for you.

<u>If it controls you, get rid of it</u>

A question I am often asked is, 'Is this food good for me?' While I have drawn a clear line in the sand between whole and processed foods, the rest of the answer is quite nuanced. Sometimes indulgences can be a positive part of your diet. But only if an occasional indulgence doesn't turn into clear abuse of food. The question that should decide whether a food is suitable in your diet or not is 'does it control you'?

Let's take chips, for instance. There's nothing wrong with some potato chips every once in a while. They're fun to eat and give you a nice psychological break from your diet. Still, when vegetables are consumed in 'chip form,' they become easy to over-consume. Can you eat a few handfuls and put the bag away, or will you end up eating the whole bag once you've started? The former person won't see any negative consequences, while the latter will suffer greatly. *What* we are indulging with is far less important than *how* we are indulging. Nut butter is my own personal example. Almond or peanut butter can be a perfectly healthy part of your diet, but not mine. If I have one tablespoon of almond or peanut butter, I will eat it until I am sick. The amount of nut butter in the house will determine my limit rather than the room in my stomach. I can't moderate rich, creamy foods. This makes spreads of all kinds unhealthy for me. That doesn't make the same true for you, but it is most definitely true for me. If a person can have a few tablespoons of tahini and put it down without issue, the food is a non-issue.

The 'can I control this' question is a consideration that is rarely made by folks when considering healthy vs. unhealthy food. Who is in control? Are you in control of the food, or is the food in control of you? It doesn't matter how healthy the food may be on paper. Overconsumption of any food is going to be an issue. While it is better to overconsume whole food than to overconsume processed junk, avoiding uncontrolled eating of any food is ideal. So you must know yourself and be realistic about what you can and can't have in your possession.

If a food controls you, you must get rid of it or risk falling victim to it. If you are in control of indulgences, you can keep less ideal foods around for the occasions when you need a 'diet break.'

A Word on 'Willpower'

When a person decides to take control of his or her diet, the first intervention usually involves willpower. We get this idea in our heads that fit people can say 'no' to foods that we always say 'yes' to. There may be some grains of truth in that idea, but we are all much more alike than you may intuit.

Willpower is a myth. The idea that getting fit means avoiding the cookies in the cupboard is an absurd concept. Human beings are evolutionarily driven to seek out high-energy, hyper-palatable foods. It is hardwired into our survival system. To focus on willpower is to work against your nature, so to push for more tremendous will as a strategy to get in shape is an often ineffective move. Get rid of foods that you can't control, and remove yourself from environments that result in binge eating and consequential consumption. At the very least, get a 'bad food box'.

Get a 'Bad Food' Box

I can't tell you how many times I've heard people complain that they can't get rid of unhealthy foods because their kids or significant other eats them. One part of me wants to say, 'well, you aren't doing your children any favors by letting them eat that crap either.' However, the more sensible part of me understands that it is hard to be responsible for other people's habits. This is when it can be a good idea to have a 'bad food box.' Every food that will remain in the house that you are likely to eat should go into a specific box or place. This is just a way to create a proper mental framework for resistance against these foods.

When we indulge in problematic foods, we often do it mindlessly or find ways to justify consumption. We rationalize why cookies are an excellent choice tonight or forget that ice cream isn't moving us closer to our goals. Putting problematic foods in a clearly marked box forces you to acknowledge that what you are about to eat will carry you away from your destination. This cognitive trick is often enough to give you the headspace necessary to change your mind about indulging. It can deliver the much-needed 'pause' between stimulus (I see food) and response (I eat the food).

So if you have kids (or adults) who make your diet a challenge with hyper-palatable foods, keep the tempting and problematic treats in a clearly marked area. That way, you can't make a choice to eat these foods without first running it by your rational brain.

In the Event of a Relapse...

Sticking to your diet is a strategy that you should aim to follow as often as possible- but you need not be so rigid that an off-track meal (or weekend) throws the whole train off the track. If you have a few glasses of red wine, a few beers, some pizza, or ice cream, you may feel like you've sabotaged all of your efforts. While I am certainly not encouraging you to eat unhealthy foods, it is silly to pretend that it's never going to happen. As I have mentioned throughout this guide- being flexible in as many ways as possible while still maintaining a general dietary structure is the key to long-term success.

I like to think of going 'off track' as taking a psychological diet break. Even though I believe you can live a very satisfying, sustainable culinary life eating whole foods, sometimes your cravings get the best of you. It is often better to allow for less nutritious foods in a controlled manner rather than avoiding them like the plague. Otherwise, you may eventually binge on junk food in a moment of stress or emotional turmoil, and the result will harm you both physically and psychologically.

You are going to go out for dinner. You are going to attend parties and functions where alcohol is free and processed foods are abundant. You may have an iron will, and if so, this section is not relevant for you. But the other 99% of the population needs a gameplan for these moments. There are ways in which you can sensibly 'indulge' in off-track eating without hindering your progress, and that is what we are going to discuss below using three key strategies.

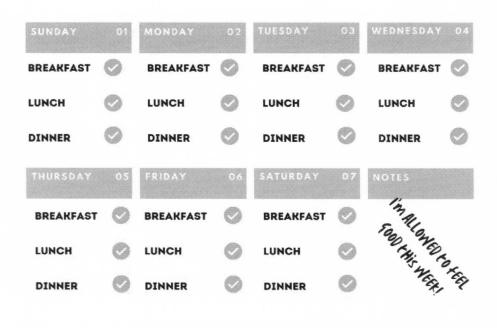

What we think success looks like.

SUNDAY 01	MONDAY 02	TUESDAY 03	WEDNESDAY 04
BREAKFAST ✓	BREAKFAST ✓	BREAKFAST ✓	BREAKFAST ✓
LUNCH ✓	LUNCH ✓	LUNCH ✓	LUNCH ✗
DINNER ✓	DINNER ✗	DINNER ✓	DINNER ✓

THURSDAY 05	FRIDAY 06	SATURDAY 07	NOTES
BREAKFAST ✓	BREAKFAST ✗	BREAKFAST ✓	*I'm SUCH A FAILURE!!!!*
LUNCH ✓	LUNCH ✓	LUNCH ✓	
DINNER ✓	DINNER ✓	DINNER ✗	

What success ACTUALLY looks like (but we usually perceive as failure)

#1 make a plan!- We overdo it when we indulge because we go into social occasions and other food events without anticipating what it will involve. We pretend not to know ourselves enough to be clear about where we are weak or where social pressures will come from. For instance, if I go to my mother's house for dinner, I know that there will be turkey, stuffing, apple pie, mashed potatoes, and alcohol! If I walked into that environment without mental planning, I would overeat and overdrink everything that came my way. We find creative ways to justify and rationalize severe abuses of food and drink when we are in the moment. However, if I make a mental note in my head of what I will allow myself to enjoy BEFORE showing up to dinner, it makes a big difference.

For example, I could say to myself, 'I will have three glasses of wine; one before dinner, one with dinner, and maybe one after dinner. I will have one small serving of mashed potatoes or stuffing, and if I am not full, I will have a small sliver of apple pie. Anything beyond that is an unreasonable indulgence'. It sounds silly, I know, but making a short mental plan of how the night will go and what you can sensibly allow yourself to enjoy will bring you a greater sense of control without having to restrict the foods you try. If you tick the mental boxes before you're in the moment, you will quickly remind yourself of what is reasonable consumption and what is not.

#2: understand the difference between food joy and food abuse- We tend to lose control while indulging in off-track eating because we justify our choices and actions in the name of 'enjoying ourselves.' I agree that there is a time to pamper yourself with food. However, I'm not sure that we all have the same definition of the word 'enjoy.' When you are genuinely enjoying yourself, you are taking small bites and experiencing specific tastes. You chew slowly and take time to think about texture. If drinking a glass of wine or a fresh beer, you take slow, small sips and taste every single ounce of your beverage. Connecting with good food and drink respectfully is the meaning of 'enjoying yourself'.

In contrast, many believe that to 'enjoy something' means that we consume large quantities until we are sick to our stomachs—more food and drink = a greater food and drink experience. Eating or drinking something you like the taste of until it makes you ill is not enjoyment; it is abuse. Abusing food and drink does not result in an increased sense of joy. Instead, it equals an increased lack of control, negative self-reflection, and consequence. If you want to enjoy yourself while indulging, slow it down. Take small bites, take small sips, savor the tastes and smells, and connect with your food and drink in a respectful way rather than an abusive one.

#3: Fill up on whole foods first and indulgences second- The order in which you consume your meals matters. Starting and finishing in the right places can make all the difference with meal control. During a family dinner or other social occasion, you should identify the low consequence and high consequence foods available and aim to first fill yourself up with the low consequence foods. Doing so will help you to control the intake of the high consequence food.

Low consequence foods have a lower caloric load compared to the nutrients and satiety that they provide. If you think back to nutrient density and the P/E ratio from earlier, these are the foods to which I am referring. Some examples would be leafy greens like lettuce, spinach, and kale. Above-ground vegetables like tomatoes, peppers, and cucumbers. Root vegetables like beets, turnips, rutabagas, and high protein foods like beef, chicken, and seafood.

High consequence foods have a higher caloric load with less nutrition, and these are the foods we tend to overeat. Some examples would be grain based carbs like bread or stuffing. High sugar condiments like cranberry sauce. Highly concentrated fats like gravy, oils, and dressings, and some fattier cuts of meat. Anything high in starch, sugar, or fat while being low in protein or nutrients qualifies as high consequence.

Once you've identified both your low and high consequence foods, aim to fill your plate with low consequence foods while mildly indulging in the high consequence foods- preferably after you've had your fill of the nutrient dense choices. Aim to consume your protein first and be liberal with your portion. Have a large salad with lots of fresh vegetables and perhaps some warm root vegetables. Once you're getting close to the point of feeling full, then you should sprinkle in some stuffing, some gravy, or a dessert option. If you go straight to the high consequence foods first, you are far more likely to overeat and add needless pounds to your body.

Mixing different foods and tastes can bypass 'palate fatigue,' the mechanism that helps prevent overeating. So if you are going back and forth from one food to another, you are much more likely to eat past satiety.

Indulging in sweet, salty, sugary, fatty, and high-calorie foods don't have to lead to guilt, shame, or pounds gained- but if you indulge in an unprepared 'free for all,' it will take an emotional and physical toll. Follow these three strategies and plan your indulgences in a controlled setting, and you can have the best of both worlds: the progress plus the pleasure!

Beware the Language of Failure

I want to conclude the book's behaviour change section with a few thoughts on how we talk to ourselves, both internally and externally. If you are used to slipping up in the past, there is a good chance you've developed a substantial vocabulary of failure. We often use the language of failure to protect us from our negative thoughts and feelings, but the constant cynical monologue prevents one from reaching their goals.

For example, when you picked up this book, you may have thought to yourself, 'this isn't likely to make any difference, but I guess I'll give it a shot'. What you are doing here is giving yourself permission to quit at any time or dismiss concepts in the book that you don't believe you can follow through on.

Perhaps while reading the section on planning for social consumption, you thought 'planning and controlling myself while out with my friends? Does this guy think I'm giving up girls' night? No way is that going to be the key to my success!' In this case, you exaggerate a suggestion that I never made so that you could tear it down and make it look silly. If it's ridiculous, you don't have to consider it a legitimate point or strategy. We use these fallacies and biases to rationalize our difficult-to-change behavior. We do so because we expect to fail. When you expect to fail, you pre-emptively create a scenario in which the failure is by-design and the fault of someone other than yourself.

I'm not critical here. This is normal human behaviour. But if you want to create an internal environment where long-term change is possible, you need to see this language for the nonsense it is and give yourself a chance to do things differently.

I encourage you to take the behaviour change section seriously. Perhaps you should consider reading it a few times and working through how these barriers show themselves in your own life. Failure is simply the accumulation of poor choices or the inability to make sound choices. Choice-making is not a matter of will or access to information. Many powerful forces have created and reinforced the negative habits that prevent us from succeeding in the long-term.

Behaviour change strategy is the only way to overcome these barriers in the long run. Without considering what is driving poor choice-making, you may be able to see success for a few months or even a year. Still, eventually, the root of your habits will come to the surface and drive you into self-sabotage, and ultimately, failure.

SUPPLEMENTATION

We finish the guide with the topic where most people want to begin: supplements. Interventions like supplementation cannot cover up your shortcomings in diet and exercise. If you aren't active every day and putting good food into your body; vitamins and minerals won't change a darn thing for you. With that being said, supplements can help you if you are already doing the foundational work in the areas of nutrition, movement, and sleep. Assuming you are doing so, here are supplements proven to benefit fat loss and muscle gain in individuals who are doing the foundational work. By 'proven,' I mean that there is robust, well-conducted research that supports the claims made by producers of these supplements.

Whey Protein: I suggest that most people get their protein from the whole foods listed in the book, but for some reason, getting adequate protein can be a struggle for people. If this is the case for you, Whey Protein can undoubtedly be helpful. Whey has been shown to significantly increase protein synthesis well beyond other supplements that have the same intended purpose. If you are Vegan, rice protein and hemp proteins with the majority of the starch removed can take the place of Whey, but plant-based alternatives are not as effective as the animal comparative. If you decide to use Whey, try not to use more than one serving of 25-40 grams per day.

I suggest no more than a single serving because you're not achieving what you need to in a whole foods diet if you are consuming more than that. The supplement's timing is much less important than the total daily protein intake, so take it when it makes sense for you.

Here is what you will find regarding Whey Protein dosage on Examine.com: *The amount of whey protein to supplement depends on individual daily protein goals. For example: If you are an athlete or highly active person attempting to lose body fat while preserving lean muscle mass, a daily intake of 1.5-2.2g/kg bodyweight (0.68-1g/lb bodyweight) is a good goal. If you are an athlete or highly active person, or you are attempting to lose body fat while preserving lean mass, then a daily intake of 1.0-1.5g/kg bodyweight (0.45-0.68g/lb bodyweight) is a good goal. If you are sedentary and not looking to change body composition, a daily target of 0.8g/kg bodyweight (0.36g/lb bodyweight) is a good goal.*

If daily protein targets are achieved through dietary protein alone, supplementation is unnecessary. Obese individuals should not follow the above recommendations, as bodyweight calculations would result in very high dosages. Obese people should calculate their protein targets based off of what their weight would be, assuming an overweight BMI.

Magnesium and Sodium: You hear about the importance of 'electrolytes' all the time, and Magnesium and Sodium are the two that most active people find themselves to be deficient in. Especially if you are on the lower end of the carbohydrate intake, these two minerals may be essential for supplementation.

Sodium is surprisingly the electrolyte that most often requires supplementation. I want to be clear that this is in active individuals who are healthy and eating well. If you spend your day sitting on your ass and eating processed food, this likely isn't the case for you. Assuming you're the former, start with 1000mgs of sodium per day (in addition to what you already take in your food). Magnesium is not something that most people eating lots of fruits and vegetables require, but magnesium supplementation is worth considering if you are more toward the 'Keto' spectrum. Begin supplementing with 100mgs per day, never going above 500mgs. Too much magnesium can cause a gastrointestinal upset in some people, so titrate slowly.

Here is what you will find about Magnesium on examine.com: *The standard dose for magnesium supplementation is 200-400mg. Any form of magnesium can be used to attenuate a magnesium deficiency, except magnesium L-threonate, since it contains less elemental magnesium per dose. Gastrointestinal side-effects, like diarrhea and bloating, are more common when magnesium oxide or magnesium chloride are supplemented, due to the lower absorption rates of these two forms. In general, magnesium citrate is a good choice for supplementation. Magnesium L-threonate can be used for cognitive enhancement. Magnesium should be taken daily, with food. Superloading magnesium, or taking more magnesium that is needed to attenuate a deficiency, should be done with magnesium diglycinate or magnesium gluconate.*

EAA's and Leucine: Essential Amino Acids and Leucine are beneficial supplements for people who want to gain significant muscle, exercise while fasting, or follow a Vegan diet. Taking EAA's of 3-5 grams while exercising fasted can help preserve muscle. Leucine is responsible for turning on muscle protein synthesis, and the average person needs to hit a threshold of 1.5-3 grams to maximize this process. Plant foods are deficient in Leucine, which is why I suggest plant based eaters utilize it. If you are a fasted exerciser, combine the two supplements and consume them throughout your fasted exercise.

If your fasted training consists of walking or something else low intensity, this isn't necessary. If you are looking to build muscle in general or supplement a plant-based diet, take the supplements when it makes the most sense for you.

This is what Examine.com has to say about Leucine: The studies assessing leucine mostly look at muscle protein synthesis when additional leucine is added to the diet or to a test meal, and it appears that leucine is able to reliably increase muscle protein synthesis after test meals.

Whether this results in more lean mass over a period of time is somewhat less reliable though, and leucine appears to be more effective at promoting gains in muscle in people with lower dietary protein intake and in the elderly (who tend to have impaired muscle protein synthesis in response to the diet). The interactions of leucine on glucose are not clear, to be honest.

Leucine possesses both blood sugar reducing properties (can release insulin from the pancreas, can directly stimulate glucose uptake into a cell without insulin) but also the opposite (via stimulating S6K, it can inhibit insulin-stimulated glucose uptake). In a cell culture, leucine stimulates glucose uptake for up to 45 minutes and then hinders itself while in living systems acute doses of leucine do not appear to do anything remarkable (some limited evidence that leucine can be rehabilitative in diabetes, but this is preliminary). Isoleucine is a more potent hypoglycemic agent, but to less inhibition of its own actions.

Vitamin D: Most of us can get enough Vitamin D in our diet if we eat enough animal foods and spend time in the sun, but that isn't what most people are doing. Especially if you live in a place with four seasons or spend your days indoors, you will want to consider taking a Vitamin D supplement for general health purposes during the darker months. Recommendations go anywhere from 400iu's to 10,000iu's daily. I believe that anywhere between 1000-3000iu's is ideal for most people. I would also suggest that you consider taking a blood test to find out your specific Vitamin D status and measure the effect of supplementation. The cost of a test is $25-$50.

This is Examine.com's take on Vitamin D: *Vitamin D is a fat-soluble nutrient. It is one of the 24 micronutrients critical for human survival. The sun is the major natural source of the nutrient, but vitamin D is also found naturally in fish and eggs. It is also added to dairy products.*

Supplemental vitamin D is associated with a wide range of benefits, including increased cognition, immune health, bone health and well-being. Supplementation can also reduce the risks of cancer, heart disease, diabetes and multiple sclerosis. People deficient in vitamin D may also experience increased testosterone levels after supplementation. The body produces vitamin D from cholesterol, provided there is an adequate amount of UV light from sun exposure. There is only a sufficient amount of UV light coming from the sun when the UV index is 3 or higher, which only occurs year-round near the equator, between the 37th parallels.

Most people are not deficient in vitamin D, but they do not have an optimal level of vitamin D either. Due to the many health benefits of vitamin D supplementation is encouraged if optimal levels are not present in the body.

Omega 3: EPA and DHA have a variety of positive effects on general health. Getting a good fish oil or Omega 3 supplement is a simple way to make sure you're getting enough of the two. One gram of EPA/DHA combined is the recommended daily dosage. That is not one gram of total fish oil or Omega 3 oil, specifically the EPA and DHA. You'll need to read the back of the bottle to find out how much of the two you get per gram/serving of oil.

This is what Examine.com has to say about Omega-3 Fish Oil: *Fish oil causes a potent reduction in triglyceride levels, and a more modest reduction in blood pressure in hypertensives.[Despite this, long-term trials haven't found a reduction in the rate of cardiovascular events.[19]*

It appears to notably improve mood in people with major depression, though it's unclear if it has an effect in people with minor depression.[20] EPA, in particular, seems to be the most effective omega-3 fatty acid for this purpose which suggests that the effects of fish oil are due to reducing neuroinflammation. Its anti-inflammatory benefits also seem to extend to reducing the symptoms of systemic lupus erythematosus. However, its benefits shouldn't be assumed to extend to inflammatory diseases in general.

Closing Thoughts

Getting in shape is not complicated. The path to peak fitness is straightforward. Eat whole foods, don't eat all day long, move often, and be sure your diet reflects your lesser energy demands when you are inactive. All other considerations in diet and exercise are unhelpful 'noise.'

We make the weight loss industry confusing for a few reasons. As professionals, you need to have a niche or an angle that makes you stand out among the millions of other coaches, trainers, and nutritionists. If there isn't some flashy magic to your approach, people are less likely to be interested in what you're selling. As consumers, we look to avoid the complex barriers between us and success. If the key to getting healthy is as simple as eating one group of foods, avoiding another group of foods, or trying fad exercises, we can avoid the truth.

The truth of the complex underlying driving forces that push us to overeat, snack late into the night, drink a little too much, and be constantly technologically distracted. We all know that increased diet and exercise information won't solve these behavioral problems, but if we hang onto the perfect diet dream, we can avoid the hard work that takes time and energy to complete. This is why we keep running on the hamster wheel of success and failure while we look for the next big trick. We try a new fad, we manage to stick to it for a few weeks or months, and we see results.

Eventually, our unaddressed habits catch up to us; we regress, self-sabotage, and then feel extreme failure, insecurity, and sadness. Frustrated and beaten down, we go back to our old ways. A few months or a few years later, we become so fed up with our growing waistlines that we look for the next 'method' to save us. Rinse, and repeat.

It is time to stop hiding behind fabulous trends, pills, cleanses, and other distractions. My goal for this book was to bring you much-needed clarity so you can get past the smoke and mirrors of the weight loss industry. I want to make dieting and fat loss simple so you can use your energy to work on the real barriers between you and success.

It is my sincere hope that reading this book starts you down the path of long-term transformation with a diet that works with you, for you, and on your terms. Anything less will push you back toward a path of negativity, frustration, and failure.

Stay positive, stay simple, and always bounce back.
Tommy

If you enjoyed this book, please consider giving it a 5 star review on Amazon. It is the best way to help me get this information into the hands of those who need it most.

REFERENCES

Protein Safety and Efficacy

https://www.ncbi.nlm.nih.gov/pmc/articles/PMC5420553/

https://www.ncbi.nlm.nih.gov/pmc/articles/PMC6491698/

https://www.ncbi.nlm.nih.gov/pmc/articles/PMC5477153/

https://www.ncbi.nlm.nih.gov/pubmed/22150425

https://academic.oup.com/advances/article/9/3/171/4964951

https://www.frontiersin.org/articles/10.3389/fnut.2019.00083/full

https://jissn.biomedcentral.com/articles/10.1186/s12970-018-0215-1

https://bjsm.bmj.com/content/52/6/376

https://www.ncbi.nlm.nih.gov/pmc/articles/PMC5078648/https://jissn.bio medcentral.com/articles/10.1186/1550-2783-11-19

https://jissn.biomedcentral.com/articles/10.1186/s12970-016-0114-2

Fasting and Time Restricted Eating for Insulin Sensitivity and Blood Glucose Control

https://jamanetwork.com/journals/jamainternalmedicine/fullarticle/262352

https://academic.oup.com/ajcn/article/81/1/69/4607679https://insights.ovi d.com/crossref?an=01938924-201802000-00016

https://www.annualreviews.org/doi/full/10.1146/annurev-nutr-071816-064634?url_ver=Z39.88-2003&rfr_id=ori%3Arid%3Acrossref.org&rfr_dat=cr_pub%3Dpubmed

https://www.sciencedirect.com/science/article/pii/S1550413118302535https://onlinelibrary.wiley.com/doi/full/10.1002/oby.22449

https://www.cell.com/cell-metabolism/fulltext/S1550-4131(19)30611-4?_returnURL=

https%3A%2F%2Flinkinghub.elsevier.com%2Fretrieve%2Fpii%2FS1550413119306114%3Fshowall%3Dtrue

https://content.iospress.com/articles/nutrition-and-healthy-aging/nha170036

Psychological Drivers of Consumption

Adam, T. C., & Epel, E. S. (2007). Stress, eating and the reward system. Physiology & Behavior, 91(4), 449-458. doi:10.1016/j.physbeh.2007.04.011

Birch, L. L., Davison, K. K., Fisher, J. O. (2003) Learning to overeat: maternal use of restrictive feeding practices promotes girls' eating in the absence of hunger. American Journal Clinical Nutrition, 78, 215–220.

Groesz, L. M., McCoy, S., Carl, J., Saslow, L., Stewart, J., Adler, N., Laraia, B., & Epel, E. (2012). What is eating you? Stress and the drive to eat. Elsevier, 58(2), 717-721. DOI: 10.1016/j.appet.2011.11.028

Herman, C. P., & Polivy, J. (2008). External cues in the control of food intake in humans: The sensory-normative distinction. Physiology & Behavior, 94(5) 722-728. doi:10.1016/j.physbeh.2008.04.014

Higgs, S. (2002). Memory for recent eating and its influence on subsequent food intake. Appetite, 39(2), 159-166. doi:10.1006/appe.2002.0500

Kandiah, J., Yake, M., Jones, J., & Meyer, M. (2006). Stress influences appetite and comfort food preferences in college women. Nutrition Research, 26(3 118-123. DOI: 10.1016/j.nutres.2005.11.010

Lambert, K.G., Neal, T., Noyes, J. et al. (1991). Current Psychology, 10, 297 303. doi:10.1007/BF02686902

Ochs, E., Pontecorva, C., & Fasulo, A. (1996). Socializing taste. Ethnos, 61(1 2). DOI:10.1080/00141844.1996.9981526

Rozin, P., Dow, S., Moscovitch, M., & Rajaram, S. (1998). What causes human to begin and end a meal? A role for memory for what has been eaten, a evidenced by a study of multiple meal eating in amnesic patients Psychological Science, 9(5), 392-396. doi:10.1111/1467-9280.00073

Rozin, P., Fischler, C., Imada, S., Sarubin, A., & Wrzesniewski, A. (1999) Attitudes to food and the role of food in life in the U.S.A., Japan, Flemish Belgium and France: Possible implications for the diet-health debate Appetite, 33(2), 163-180. doi:10.1006/appe.1999.0244

Schachter, S. (1968). Obesity and eating. Science, 161(3843), 751-756 doi:10.1126/science.161.3843.751

artanian, L. R., Wansink, B., & Herman, C. P. (2008). Are We Aware of the xternal Factors That Influence Our Food Intake? Health Psychology, 27(5), 33-538. Doi: 10.1037/0278-6133.27.5.533

Sleep, Stress, and Weight Management

https://www.nih.gov/news-events/nih-research-matters/molecular-ties-between-lack-sleep-weight-gain

https://www.sciencedaily.com/releases/2006/05/060529082903.htmhttps:/advances.sciencemag.org/content/4/8/eaar8590

https://jamanetwork.com/journals/jamainternalmedicine/article-abstract/2735446

https://www.newswise.com/articles/losing-30-minutes-of-sleep-per-day-may-promote-weight-gain-and-adversely-affect-blood-sugar-control

https://www.uchicagomedicine.org/forefront/news/sleep-loss-limits-fat-loss

https://www.sciencedaily.com/releases/2019/04/190425143610.htmhttp://med.stanford.edu/news/all-news/2018/04/timing-of-stress-hormone-pulses-controls-weight-gain.html

https://www.ucsf.edu/news/2011/12/11091/stress-reduction-and-mindful-eating-curb-weight-gain-among-overweight-women

https://msutoday.msu.edu/news/2015/childhood-stress-fuels-weight-gain-in-women/

https://www.sciencedaily.com/releases/2000/11/001120072314.htm

Supplement Safety, Efficacy, and Dosage

Whey Protein: https://examine.com/supplements/whey-protein/

Creatine: https://examine.com/supplements/creatine/

EAA's: https://examine.com/topics/essential-amino-acids/

Leucine: https://examine.com/supplements/leucine/

Vitamin D: https://examine.com/supplements/vitamin-d/

EPA/DHA (Fish Oil): https://examine.com/supplements/krill-oil/

Magnesium: https://examine.com/supplements/magnesium/

Made in the USA
Monee, IL
21 December 2020